The Skin Cure Diet

The Skin Cure Diet

✦

Heal Eczema from Inside Out

Kathleen Waterford

iUniverse, Inc.
New York Lincoln Shanghai

The Skin Cure Diet
Heal Eczema from Inside Out

Copyright © 2005 by Kathleen Waterford

iUniverse books may be ordered through booksellers or by contacting:

iUniverse
2021 Pine Lake Road, Suite 100
Lincoln, NE 68512
www.iuniverse.com
1-800-Authors (1-800-288-4677)

ISBN-13: 978-0-595-35883-0 (pbk)
ISBN-13: 978-0-595-80340-8 (ebk)
ISBN-10: 0-595-35883-7 (pbk)
ISBN-10: 0-595-80340-7 (ebk)

Printed in the United States of America

Contents

Chapter 1 Purpose: Who May Benefit 1

Chapter 2 Symptoms: Elusive and Ever-Changing 3

Chapter 3 Case Study: My Story 5

Chapter 4 Yeast Infection Connection 18

Chapter 5 Diet Evolution and Inflammatory Statements 20

Chapter 6 The Diet and Recovery: Stages and Timing 23

Chapter 7 Week 1: Preparing for the Diet 24

Chapter 8 Week 2 to 5: The Diet 26

Chapter 9 The Diet: Foods to Eat and Avoid 29

Chapter 10 Recipes 32

Chapter 11 Week 6: Evaluate, Ease Off the Diet, and Curb
Inflammation 37

Chapter 12 Maintenance, Supplements and Tips 39

Appendix Internet Resources 41

1

Purpose: Who May Benefit

I decided to write this after discovering that my life-long, severe eczema came from *inside*, not outside as I had always heard and read.

It was *not* caused by too much sunlight, or too little; wearing wool clothing; or even by scratching (don't the doctors who cite scratching itself as a cause ever wonder where the itch came from in the first place? It came from *inside*).

I discovered, to my shock, that I do *not* have to slather my entire body with cortisone creams and moisturizers every morning and night just to be able to move.

It was just as I always sensed intuitively, and I remember telling doctors and my parents this when I was little, but I just couldn't articulate it and, of course, had no idea of what the specifics were anyway.

The goal of this guide is to help people with almost any kind of skin disorder heal themselves without ongoing dependence on drugs, creams, lotions, or other medicines by relating what worked for me to cure my eczema, dermatitis and acne. There's a lot of information out there, especially on the internet, but much of it seems vague or conflicting regarding the combination of symptoms I had. If you've had no luck with doctors, allergy drugs, cortisone cream, or other eczema treatments, this particular combination of treatments that I stumbled upon may also help you.

Not only is there contradictory advice on eczema in literature and online, but I've also heard it from the many doctors I've seen for years for dry skin, eczema, dermatitis, candida, asthma and food allergies, from New York to California to Canada. They're trying to help, but there just does not seem to be enough conclusive research on skin conditions yet, so they end up passing on bits and pieces of information that, at least for me, never added up to a complete picture of health until I took matters into my own hands and created a skin cure diet plan for myself.

1

I did a lot of informal research and trial and error over a long period of time and eventually I cured my skin's health, overall health, and most of my allergies with a natural diet, natural antibiotics, anti-inflammatories and anti-fungals to fight candida albicans. Candida is a yeast infection, which in my case was on the surface of the skin, and just under it, subcutaneously. It was like having athlete's foot migrate to different parts of your body, putting extra stress on your general health and causing various types of skin and other health conditions.

Please note: I'm not a health professional. I've personally experienced a full range of painful and severe rashes and allergies for almost forty years, tried every treatment until I hit upon the right combination of diet, exercise and lifestyle for me, so I want to pass it on in the hope that it will work for others as well—especially for children so they can get into good health habits at an early age. I'm hoping to share the experience, but not to advise: your doctor should be consulted for that, and before making any significant changes in your diet or health lifestyle.

Speaking of other aspects of your health, I found this diet also cured my acne, which I used to get twice monthly, right on schedule with ovulation and my period (now I've only had two pimples in the past six months, and they were practically invisible); migraine headaches for which I used to have to take Fiorinol, which is a narcotic (and am now completely off that); and as a bonus I lost the ten extra pounds I had hanging around.

I will describe the diet, the steps I went through in changing my lifestyle, the websites, food, products, and other resources I used, the stages of recovery, tips and maintenance.

2

Symptoms: Elusive and Ever-Changing

The symptoms I had were also, not coincidentally I believe, many of the ones most often cited as being attributable to candida yeast overgrowth. They also had a habit of coming and going without warning, no apparent pattern, and with one apparently replacing the other over time.

- eczema: blistering, weeping, peeling, red flaky skin

- dermatitis: dry, sensitive, itchy skin rash (as opposed to the wet nature of eczema)

- hands and feet: blisters and red, scaly patches on my palms and soles

- swelling (edema) on the face: puffy eyelids, lips, ears, and scalp

- oral thrush: red mouth and lips, bad breath, drooling on the pillow while sleeping

- hair loss: itchy, burning scalp, or sometimes just dandruff and mild soreness

- more hair loss: even from my eyebrows, eyelashes and arms

- eyes: burning, very sensitive to light

- swollen, painful joints: especially ankles, knees, hands, elbows

- severe muscle aches, where it feels like it's actually the bone that's hurting

- hives (urticaria): popping up in different areas on the body

- inflamed fingernails and toenails, peeling along the sides and cuticles

- extreme fatigue: often sleeping two or three hours more per night than usual. I've also seen this aptly described as a feeling of "trying to walk through molasses"

- varying effects of diet on your skin and mood with no apparent rhyme or reason

- brain fog: mild but chronic dizziness, short attention span, impatience for details, moodiness, an odd sort of surreal feeling of detachment from my life

- menstrual problems: severe PMS and cramps; flaring up of symptoms even during ovulation

- allergies: apparently allergen-triggered hay fever; sneezing when around pets; my mouth and throat breaks out in hives if I have peanuts, eggs or dairy products

- cigarette smoke sensitivity: just one breath of second hand smoke made me dizzy and wheezy; probably my most extreme allergy besides peanuts

- migraine headaches: the kind that come with light-sensitivity and extreme nausea to the point where I couldn't eat for a day

I rarely had all these symptoms at once while growing up, but they kept building while rotating themselves, once after another, until I reached three health crisis points that I describe in the next chapter.

3

Case Study: My Story

Childhood

I'll go into some detail regarding my background so that you can see if it matches your situation or that of your child. I had the typical allergic child's early experiences. Apparently when I was a baby, I had very sensitive digestion, reacting poorly to various foods, had frequent ear infections, insomnia and cried a lot. My mother, a nurse, says she breast-fed me a few months longer than whatever the standard was in the 1960's and that that seemed to help. This is consistent with recent studies recommending longer breast-feeding for all children to even help prevent allergies before they take root in the baby. There is something about the transference of immunologic cells from the mother that bolsters the baby's immune system.

The eczema started when I was about three years old. That was my earliest memory of having a dysfunctional immune system. The characteristic red, itchy blisters appeared on my right heel first (and, coincidentally—or maybe not such a coincidence—that was the last place to heal when I finally got well 36 years later).

Of course it was downhill from there: I'm sure anyone who had a similar type of skin disorder in childhood, or has gone through the parenting of one, is all too familiar with the domino and cyclical effect. The shoes rub against the blister, it starts weeping making the surrounding area itchier; the child scratches that area, spreading it and opening it up to infection; it gets infected and gets itchier.

The vicious cycle continues with the recommendations that still appear to exist today: hydrocortisone creams, various medicinal, oatmeal or tar bath treatments, and antihistamines. The problem I found is that sometimes those things made it better, but more often it became worse or stayed the same. Usually I considered it a good day if I woke up and it wasn't worse than it was the day before.

The effects of the emotional vicious cycle are strong too. The itching and scratching can keep the child awake until late into the night. If the child can't get enough sleep, he probably won't be in as good a mood as he otherwise would.

His mood will suffer and won't get along so well with friends or school. The pain and stinging of the surface of the skin, right where so many nerves are, can be hard to manage: many days I couldn't go to school because the pain was so bad.

Bathing itself became a pain management tool. I found that extremely hot water would numb it long enough that after the initial, inevitable stinging effect, I would have a nice thirty-minute vacation from the pain. Sometimes more. I knew this would dry it out more later, but it was worth it to get this temporary alleviation. Besides which, when I would try a shorter bath, it's not like the eczema went away or would even be noticeably better—it would just be a little bit less dry. A shower used to sting too much: I guess it was the effect of the air plus the water that would do that. My skin had to be fully immersed. (I have only recently been able to tolerate showers instead of baths). Adding oatmeal preparations or baking soda did seem to help sometimes, but because it would never actually cure it, and because the alleviation would be so slight, I often found it more trouble than it was worth as I got older.

By the time I was six or seven years old, the doctors were well along the way to ascertaining that I had severe allergies. The problem was that that knowledge didn't help me get better: it didn't change anything. My parents took me to specialists in the fields of dermatology, allergies and immunology; I had the full range of skin tests; I had weekly allergy shots for years against hay fever and pet dander—they never seemed to be effective, although consistency is important for these types of shots, and I was never well enough for more than two weeks in a row to be able to receive them. Not well enough to go to the doctor's office! But my skin kept gradually getting worse. We tried having me in a "dust-free" environment, but that's hard to keep up, especially since both my parents worked. We couldn't find anything that worked well or consistently, and the doctors told me there was no known cure.

Little bouts of childhood stresses and traumas would bring out the eczema too: it didn't seem to cause, but would definitely aggravate it. For instance, at five years old I had some slight blistering a red itchiness on the inside of my right wrist, and as soon as I started kindergarten, it became so bad within the first month that to this day I can see the white marks, from losing the pigmentation there, in the shape of three fingers from my left hand scratching it. The coloring is also gone from the worst areas of my ankles, knees, fingers, back, and elbows. I used to think they were scars, but a doctor told me that technically they're not: it's just irreversible pigmentation loss. I don't mind so much, except when I'm out in the sun and the rest of my body tans while these areas stay bright white.

But in a way I like it, since it reminds me that these areas have healed, and having healthy white skin there is much better than what used to be there.

Another factor that had surfaced was asthma. I didn't have a severe case, as far as I could tell. I had light wheezing when I had a cold. But at least part of the problem was that both my parents smoked, so it appeared that I had developed a harsh allergy to cigarettes. It was only just becoming known at that time how toxic this was.

One possible effect of this was the fact that I had many severe bouts with pneumonia growing up. I was hospitalized for two of them, when I was three and five. It was the oxygen tent and the antibiotics and the wheezing and more antibiotics: the whole thing. Lots of coughing up of mucus for weeks at a time and lots of school missed. I took physical therapy for asthma while in the hospital, and the main treatment was just trying to inhale deeply and hold it. A simple thing, but it worked well. This helped show me the effectiveness of something natural, non-medical. The main problem with the asthma is that it just added another huge load to my immune system—and the mass quantities of antibiotics I consumed will be an important point in a later chapter when we discuss the actual diet.

(I keep reading in the newspapers that the incidence of asthma has been increasing for children, especially in urban centers, and that it's a mystery as to what factors might be causing this. I believe that it's directly linked to diet, rather than air pollution, dust and other airborne allergens, as a few of the theories that have been offered up but unproven. It would be a good idea for someone to test the effects of diet on the asthma conditions of these poor kids, since we know diet is one variable that has drastically changed for the worse in the past twenty years—unlike air quality, which has actually improved).

So my overall symptoms and condition by about age eight, and corresponding treatments, were Intal powder inhaler on a regular basis (I think it was four times a day) and Ventolin inhaler for emergencies; frequent antibiotics, usually Erythromycin, for pneumonia, other various bronchial infections, and skin infections; antihistamines occasionally for hay fever, which was also not too severe; hydrocortisone creams and lotions for the skin rashes, which concentrated mostly on my face, neck and joints, especially the ankles, backs and fronts of knees and elbows, and wrists; and Atarax, Benadryl, and Gravol medicine to help me with the insomnia.

Back to the vicious cycle: the drugs, even the antihistamines back then, which was in the days prior to the advent of non-drowsy medicine, made me feel dopey and non-responsive at school, so I wouldn't take them very often: maybe two or three times per week. And, of course, when I would take them consistently on a regular basis, I would notice that they would lose their effectiveness gradually after a week or two had passed, so I would have to increase the dosage to get the same effect.

The one drug that was often recommended for me, but then always decided against, was Prednisone. As you probably know, this is cortisone by mouth, in tablet form. Apparently this had been a popular treatment in the 1950s for almost any kind of inflammation, but by the '60s and '70s there were serious side effects to note. Since it suppresses inflammation by suppressing the immune system, it could make one more vulnerable to illnesses other than the one you're trying to cure. There could also be severe bloating, liver and kidney toxicity, and stunting of bone growth and therefore not suitable for children at all.

So by the time I was eleven or twelve, my parents and I had for the most part given up on the conventional medical treatments. I was still applying cortisone creams, but they seemed to be just barely keeping the eczema outbreaks in check, rather than helping to heal them. There seemed to be nothing new under the sun with the doctors and the state of the latest research, and as I was becoming more of a mouthy and belligerent preteen, I usually refused my mother's urgings to go see them.

We were still under the mistaken impression that the root of all my problems was allergies. Allergies that I genetically inherited, and were therefore fixed, and so there was nothing we could do about them.

Teenager: Sensing the Food Connection

My biggest problems by the time I reached age twelve were that I was chubby, had the full set of railroad track orthodontic braces on my smile, and very thick lenses on my eye glasses. I had accepted my skin outbreaks as a way of life and they were generally eclipsed by the more usual teenage concerns. I was more worried about the clusters of pimples I would get on my face rather than the fact that almost every one of my joints had an unattractive, itchy, red rash with thick scabs. At least I could cover those up with clothes. I was quite thankful to be living in the Pacific Northwest climate for that reason.

One interesting ray of hope occurred when I was twelve. Looking back now, I wish I could've picked up on this sooner—but better in my thirties than never. During the summer I hung out with friends who were much more active than I was. I started walking around more, riding a bike and going to the beach. This squeezed out a lot of the time that I had previously spent eating. And since it was summer, I was eating lighter, healthier fare anyway: more produce, and we were catching our own fish—salmon—and eating that regularly.

I didn't even notice that I was losing weight until it was time to leave the summer cottage, go back to the suburbs, back to school and to a regular physical checkup at the doctor's. He noted that I had lost weight even though I had grown significantly taller. And as a side note, we could all see that the state of my skin was the best we could ever remember it being.

Yet even then, no one made the connection between diet, increased activity, and my eczema. As far as I remember, it wasn't even discussed other than to perhaps assume that my generally improved health had some mysterious kind of positive effect on my skin. Other than that, it seemed to be regarded as pure coincidence.

Unfortunately, when I started school again, with its usually stresses and easy availability of foods like cookies and cake, I started gaining weight again. I became unhappy about that and noticed my skin was getting worse: itchier, and it seemed to be spreading. It was also entering the age of acne, in full swing. It was harder to sleep at night, which again set off the vicious cycle that I had in early childhood. Less sleep, feeling worse at school, getting every cold, flu and bronchitis that came along, missing more school, feeling isolated, more moodiness, hormones fluctuating. These factors made the real ones that much harder to pin down, so we attributed my worsening skin conditions to my apparently weak immune system combined with the normal teenage stressors and biological changes.

After a few more years of this, I started to become interested in a course in biology when I was fifteen. Luckily by then, I could handle more advanced reading material, so I started reading up on the subject of allergies. I was trying to figure out how I could decrease the level of immunoglobulin E, or IgE, in my system, which apparently is one of the key factors in determining a person's level of allergic sensitivity. But then I realized that there's probably nothing so complex about my situation. In reading over and over about how milk and other dairy products was one of the most common allergens, I started to wonder how badly they might be affecting me.

The problem with allergies is that they bring out such varied reactions: when I was a child and would accidentally bite into a cookie that contained peanuts, just one bite would cause my lips to puff up in hives and my throat to practically close; yet when I had milk or cheese or ice cream, sometimes I would get a stinging feeling or slight puffiness to my lips and a strange burning sensation in my throat—yet sometimes nothing, it would be fine.

I read that that is the kind of mask that allergies can hide behind, and that it's especially true if your body is constantly being overwhelmed by a certain substance. I would only have peanuts very occasionally: by accident maybe once every 4 years or so. But like every kid, I was consuming some kind of dairy product in some form every day. All the reading I was doing seemed to indicate that it takes at least five days for a food to leave your digestive system and blood stream.

So I tried abstaining from milk for five days. It was hard, especially when I realized how much dairy there is in products that I would never think of: bread, hot dogs, even some brands of canned tuna! I became a vigilant reader of food labels.

Sure enough, when I introduced in back into my diet a few days later, my lips hived up more than it ever had previously from milk, my throat burned and swelled and my stomach felt like it was bloating to about three times its size from just one glass of milk.

That convinced me to cut it out of my diet. The problem with that was: it was hard to let go. Maybe it's because I was still a teen and it was now a forbidden item, even though self-imposed. I may have been compelled by and attracted to the apparent danger. But I would still slip up, or feel the need to experiment to see if I was *still* allergic to it, every few weeks. I couldn't face the idea of never having pizza or ice cream again: it seemed like a prison sentence. This was in the time before there were the non-dairy alternatives that are so prevalent in health food stores, and even regular grocery stores, today.

The effect on my skin was very good: the rashes stopped spreading, seemed reasonably contained, and some patches cleared up when I wasn't consuming dairy. But when I would try it again, the skin problems flared up and would stay very stubbornly for a couple of weeks, at least. It wouldn't clear up completely, but at least it improved. One of the most noticeable effects was the dramatic decrease in the painfulness of my joints and the overall surface of my skin.

That made me think about what other things I might be allergic to that I could cut out. Cigarette smoke was the next big one on my list, and at least it wasn't a food. My mom had given up smoking with I was about twelve when she had a suspected lung problem, but my dad found it too hard to give up. It permeated all areas of the house. Luckily, when I was sixteen, we moved to a house with a den that had French doors, so he smoked only in there. I immediately noticed an improvement in my ability to breathe!

I can't say the decrease in my exposure to smoke had a big effect on my skin, but I did feel better overall. One things tends to lead to another when you're doing healthy things (just like when you're doing unhealthy things), and my increased oxygen apparently made me want more, so I started walking regularly. I would walk three miles home from school, where I used to take the bus. This was the first time I was getting any significant exercise since the one summer when I was outdoors a lot and eating lightly. Again, I don't recall that my skin got better, and in fact the heavy walking when I was wearing shoes and socks made the eczema on my feet worse, so I walked only every other day in order to give my skin one day to rest and heal a bit. But it made me feel so much better in general, catching fewer colds and especially fewer bronchial ones and no more of my previously biannual bout of pneumonia, that I kept doing it until I finished high school and went to college.

Twenties: Healing by Accident

College was actually easier for me than high school, since there was less time spent in the classroom and more flexible free time. I arranged my classes such that most of them were on Mondays, Wednesday, and Fridays, so if I was sick I could try to only miss Tuesdays and Thursdays and not miss too many classes.

I was still walking, and still struggling with my diet and with avoiding dairy, but by the time I was twenty I was well enough to move into the college dorm. I felt that I had missed out on a lot of socializing in high school from being sick and saw this as a great opportunity to catch up, by just plunging myself in, dorm cafeteria and all. The good news by then about my eczema was that it was quite contained to a few areas: these areas were particularly strong and stubborn, but still I could hide them most of the time (never, ever, was I not wearing socks in public). I finished college with my health at about the same place I started, so at least it had stabilized.

In my later twenties, I was working and living on my own, and was in the midst of the pasta craze of the early 1990s. I was carbohydrate-loading along with everyone else, and loving it: a little too much. I was still a good fifteen to twenty pounds overweight, which may not sound like much, but I think it is when you're young, have a small frame and you're not in great health. I think it's too much of a load for the body to efficiently handle. And the weight was creeping up as I continued to have a huge heaping bowl of pasta or rice for dinner every night, which maybe a little meat and vegetables thrown in. I was still diligent about avoiding dairy, but I was also avoiding all fats and oils since I understood them to be the enemy.

I was into that kind of diet throughout my late twenties, and at the same time my health was deteriorating. My eczema was getting worse: not just in the usual joints and creases areas, but also spreading to new parts it had never been before. It appeared in a fine, red rash all over my arms, legs, back and neck. So, basically, all over. For some reason my face was usually spared, but it often looked bloated, with dark circles under my eyes, which I had also had during my sickest periods of childhood.

The other two biggest symptoms I had were insomnia and migraine headaches. The migraines started when I was twenty-five. I recall that the day before I got it I was PMS, had a fight with my boyfriend, was stressed at work, and consumed a huge amount of chocolate. I knew this type of headache was different than any type I had previously had, since it came with blinding lights and shadowy vision, extreme nausea and a searing pain on one half of my head for twelve hours, then moved to the other half for twelve, then was suddenly over as suddenly as it began, after my period started.

I wasn't sure what was causing my insomnia, but assumed it was mostly because my skin condition had been getting worse, and the spread of the rash meant that I was always itchy somewhere. The itching would wake me up in the middle of the night, so even when I was able to fall asleep, it was often interrupted and fitful. I had successfully avoided taking any medication for quite a few years. I rarely even took a painkiller for cramps or the headaches because it always seemed that my skin would erupt into a horrible state two or three days after taking any drug. But the lack of sleep was really wearing on me, and I'm sure it was adding to another vicious cycle that was like the one from my childhood: lack of sleep leading to lower immunity, getting more colds, missing school (I was working full time and trying to take post-graduate courses at night); crying at the drop of a hat; eating more to console myself; feeling bloated and cranky; and getting itchier.

Finally one day I woke up and I could hardly move. My joints were dead stuff. My skin was so painful all over that my eyes were watering just from the stinging of it. I went to the family doctor, to whom I had been a few times before, but usually just for the flu or a sore throat, for which he would give me antibiotics. I had seen him and a dermatologist in the previous few years for my skin, but still the story was that it couldn't be cured, there was no new helpful research, and the best they could do was to prescribe antibiotics when my skin looked more infected than usual. I was probably on antibiotics two or three times a years during my twenties.

On this occasion, he said that I had some kind of systemic inflammation of the eczema, so the usual cortisone creams would be no use. He prescribed Prednisone, oral cortisone which I had never taken. I was very hesitant, but was willing to try anything and at this point, since I was so much older, I of course wasn't as worried about the side effects that might affect a child more than an adult.

So I started Prednisone for the first time in my life, at age twenty-eight, and it was like a miracle. The lighter rash areas cleared up with two days—and almost all the stubborn areas, like my ankles, healed within four. I couldn't believe it: I was almost in shock. I had never seen these parts of me be normal. And even though I knew that the Prednisone was temporary, and that I'd have to taper off, it proved to me that my skin *could* be normal. I always just assumed, subconsciously I think, that it was a permanent disability, like missing limbs. I knew then it could be cured, but wasn't sure how, and wasn't sure whether this *was* the cure or not. But I was so happy that I didn't care much at that point.

I was so happy, in fact, that I was motivated to become healthier in other areas as well. I started to feel more attractive, so that encouraged me to eat healthier and to exercise more. One thing led to another, just like the opposite of the vicious cycles from childhood. I lost fifteen pounds quickly and easily, which I was surprised about since I had read that one of the side effects from cortisone was weight gain and bloating.

I tapered off but didn't go completely off it by the time two or three months had passed. I would go off it for a few days, but then any slight flare-up would scare me, so I would take small dosages: maybe ten milligrams the first day, and five each for a couple of days after that.

In the meantime, emotionally, I was feeling the happiest I'd been in a long time. I had good friends and dated fairly regularly, but I knew that my social skills weren't at their best due to all the school I missed and social occasions I passed up when I wasn't feeling well or didn't feel like exposing my skin. So I decided to move to New York City, which I had visited on vacation a couple of times in the past and loved it, to catch up on my career, socialization, culture, and just for the challenge of it. I was eating light by the time I arrived there, and my skin was mostly healed—but it hadn't yet healed completely, and I was still using the cortisone as a crutch.

Thirties: Research and Relapse

The first year I was in New York was stressful, of course, and my diet gradually became worse as did my skin. I started eating more fast food and more bread products, especially bagels, and Chinese food. I got through the initial first three years fairly well, and attributed my worsening skin to stress, using the cortisone I had saved from my initially large prescriptions to get me through the worst periods, but I was running out and it didn't seem as effective anymore anyway, so I soon stopped taking it completely. I was focusing more on my work, so that helped me be in denial about my skin, and it had localized itself back to mainly just my joint areas, so it was easier to hide.

The migraines came back too, so I went to a doctor for that: he said that now that I was in my early thirties, my estrogen levels were plummeting like a rock, and that was what was triggering the headaches. It was true that I could anticipate a PMS headache every month like clockwork. He gave me a prescription for Fiorinol, which was the only thing that seemed to work, though like other drugs it seemed to set off my skin a few days after taking it.

The next crisis occurred after I moved into a new apartment in the city and decided to spray it with insecticide myself. Again, and it's not like I can prove that this triggered it, but the next day it felt like my skin had hardened, like it was encased in a painful suit of armor, and it was even somewhat wet all over, like tiny bubbles bursting. This time I didn't want to take cortisone because I figured I had already had enough of that, and besides, the last times I had taken it, it had seemed ineffective. So I read up on natural methods of detoxification, went to health food stores, and decided to cleanse my system. I went vegetarian, wheat-free, sugar-free, was still dairy-free, and for the first time started taking cleansing herbs like milk thistle. It took about three months, but finally the worst of it was over and I had lost weight that had built up.

Encouraged again, I became skinnier than ever: a size zero, which I didn't even know existed until I became one. For most of my childhood and into my twenties, I was a size twelve. I was eating healthy foods and a lot of soy. My skin was better—but still, not to repeat myself but this point is important: it would not clear up completely, no matter what I tried. And after years in the big city, I decided it was time to get out of there and the polluted environment. I had been traveling back and forth to California for work, had made some friends there, so that's where I decided to move.

I had the movers pick up my stuff on September 10, 2001. I was going to go to Europe for two weeks starting the next day, while my furniture was being transported to California. So I ended up waking up on September 11 to the shock of the World Trade Center crisis with just an air mattress, laptop, and radio. Of course I scrapped my plans and just headed straight to California as soon as I could.

My health was stable for the first few months there, and I was well enough to go hiking, but at six months I was worse than ever. Not only was my skin worse and the headaches returned, but I had other strange new symptoms like extreme sensitivity to light. Not only did it hurt my eyes, but it seemed to even hurt my skin when exposed to it: even artificial light, not just sunlight. I was so fatigued that I was sleeping over ten hours on some days, and could just not get out of bed. My hair was thinning rapidly—I seemed to be shedding everywhere. I realized I had not been eating well since I moved, and had been eating lots of baked goods, and things like pie baked with artificial sweetener instead of sugar to try to keep myself sugar-free.

Realization and Recovery

I wondered if I had chronic fatigue syndrome, lupus, a thyroid condition, or cancer. I seemed to have elements of those, but didn't entirely fit their descriptions, and then there was the overriding element of the eczema, which was clearly the worst problem. I kept applying over the counter cortisone creams with minimal effect, and I still didn't want to take it internally. In addition, my childhood asthma had come back and I had all kinds of digestion problems.

What helped differentiate it and identify it this time were the strange new symptoms (which I list in detail in the Symptoms chapter). Thank goodness for the advent of the internet and keyword search technology. I kept plugging in new terms and reading for a couple of days, trying to keep an open mind and not just search for allergy or skin-related illnesses like I always had before.

Finally I hit upon "yeast infection"—that kept popping up on my screen. I kept dismissing thinking, "I never get yeast infections," until I read that it can be on the skin. What really struck me were not only the long list of symptoms that matched, but also the causes: antibiotic use, the more the worse (and I had had a lot); cortisone, low protein diets, any severely restrictive diets, stress, and eating foods you're allergic to. That all fit my case perfectly.

So I went to a health food store and bought an anti-yeast diet supplement, all natural, and went on the diet that came included in the instructional brochure. No carbohydrates for three weeks! No grains, no soy! I couldn't believe, since those had been the focus of my diet for years. Even though I was usually low on wheat, I countered that with lots of rice and oatmeal.

But I tried it because now I had a new enemy: the eczema had finally spread to my face. My eyelids and ears were peeling, my scalp was burning and flaky, and my neck was red and hivy. My face was generally bloated and painful. Looking back, I'm glad that happened, or I might not have had the motivation to take this new diet seriously without this hit to my vanity. The face is hard to hide. I had been able to avoid many things before in my diet: no dairy for years, no eggs, no wheat, no meat—but never had I tried eating just fish, poultry and vegetables. Never, not even for one meal, I'm sure—let alone for three weeks.

I started the diet and the supplements, stopped taking any medication and even cortisone cream, and after three days it got worse. Luckily, I had read that that might happen, so I persisted. After the three weeks were up, the pain had mostly gone, the itchiness had gone, my skin looked better—but still not great. I thought, "oh well" and added back some brown rice foods and grapefruit, like the diet plan suggested. Then, for some reason and I'm not sure why, maybe because I hadn't used any cortisone cream for awhile, I put a thin layer all over one night after a bath. And by the end of the next day, my skin was virtually perfect.

I really couldn't believe it. I stopped applying the cortisone, expecting it to come back. I kept up with the general maintenance lo-carb diet. And my skin just completely cleared up. This time, *all* areas were healed, not just some, and not just some bad patches migrating and spreading to other areas.

That's when I realized what I really had: a system-wide yeast infection, also known as candidiasis after the yeast called candida albicans, plus inflammation that didn't know when to stop. When the underlying condition of the fungal infection was gone, and an anti-inflammatory applied, it only then had a chance to take effect.

That was three years ago: since then, my skin stayed perfectly clear, and I mean 99% clear with only the occasional PMS itch, for two full years. Not only that, but I lost weight healthfully, eating a natural diet and I haven't had a migraine in three years. I no longer get the monthly acne outbreak, PMS in general is hardly noticeable, my hair grew back fuller than it was before, my hay fever is gone, and even the skin on my face that never had eczema looks better. I had creases on my forehead that are now barely visible and the rest of my face looks so good, that it can't be a coincidence that within a year of completing the diet I was ID'd twice, once at a club and once at a grocery store even under those bright lights—and even though I was in my late thirties!

Like before, though, I felt compelled to test fate, and after two years of success I started eating foods I had previously avoided, like dairy, eggs and wheat. I thought, "how do I know for sure that it was candida? Maybe it was just the move to California that helped me recover, maybe I just grew out of it, or maybe it was just a fluke." And guess what: even though it appeared that at first I could tolerate all the foods, I relapsed after six months and the eczema came back all over, just as bad as it ever was. I went back on the diet, but the supplements I took the first time didn't seem to work, so I went to stronger ones (which I describe in the diet). It worked eventually, thank goodness again, but took longer. I also went to an immunologist, who gave me allergy tests and it turned out I was very allergic to dairy, eggs, wheat and soy, which I had been eating a lot of in every form: soy milk, soy butter, soy ice cream, etc. Now I completely stay away from all of those.

This made me decide to *never* underestimate this condition again, to eat a plain and nutritious diet, avoid all allergens, and to write this all down so that other people can share and hopefully benefit from my mistakes and success.

4

Yeast Infection Connection

I wondered why my patches of eczema seemed mostly to be in the creases: the insides of my elbows, knees and ankles.

Then one day, when my skin was at its worst, as I described in my story, I just kept scanning all the websites I could find, using variety of keyword combinations that weren't like the typical ones I previously searched to find information on eczema. I used to use the obvious ones like "dry skin," "dermatitis," and "allergies," but then I decided to attack it sideways by trying more descriptive phrases of the actual symptoms. There were some symptoms that seemed so unique and paradoxical to me, like the fact that when my skin would flare up, I would often become very sensitive to light at the same time.

I was shocked and in a certain state of denial initially when the same verdict kept appearing on the screen: "candida overgrowth," also known as a just plain "yeast infection"—even "athlete's foot." It lives and thrives in the creases of skin of susceptible individuals, where the darkness and dampness help it survive.

How could that be? I *never* got yeast infections! And I am certainly no athlete. In almost forty years I had only had one vaginal yeast infection—and that was in college so I figured it can hardly count. But at least I had that one experience that defined for me that fact that I knew I had never had another one.

But it turns out that the yeast can migrate anywhere in the body, creating chaos and obscure, vague symptoms that are hard to specifically attach to any one disease or condition. In my case, and again, I'm not a doctor, so this is all from my experience, not my own formal medical research, but I believe I had a yeast infection all over my skin, either just under it, on top of it, or both.

Not much is officially know about it because it is so difficult to study: yeast is there naturally in the body since birth, and it is hard to quantify, so it's hard to know when there's an overgrowth. The overgrowth of the "bad" yeast versus the "good," and the toxins they release, are what cause the symptoms, and this growth is fueled by sugar, starches, low immunity and other factors including:

- use of even *one* course of antibiotics *ever*—though the more courses, and more recently, the worse: this facilitates the buildup of yeast

- use of steroids, especially cortisone, and aspirin

- taking birth control pills

- being pregnant, or any kind of hormonal imbalance

- intense stress or trauma

- significant change in life circumstance, like moving to a different climate

- a low-protein, high carbohydrate diet

- any immune deficiency for a significant period of time

- digestive problems, especially constipation, keeps the fungus in your system

- alcohol and smoking

- environmental pollutants and molds, which help feed the yeast

- a damp environment

How many of these factors have affected you in the past two years, or in the two years immediately preceding the time you started to feel seriously ill? Apparently that is the key amount of time it takes for yeast to gain a foothold in your system and drag you down. I experienced almost all of the above, especially the antibiotics exposure. Usually, most people know to take yogurt to restore the friendly flora that is killed off after a dose of antibiotics—but I never did that because I was allergic to milk. Then, when soy yogurt was developed, I tried to avoid that too because of the sugar. If I had know then what I know now about the seriousness and insidiousness of yeast, I would have taken acidophilus capsules (described later in the book) and cut back on all carbs for a few weeks.

5

Diet Evolution and Inflammatory Statements

For years I was a vegetarian and felt healthy. I lost weight and my digestion felt lighter. But I'm not sure that I was doing it correctly, as I also sometimes felt bloated, had worse eczema during the end of this period, headaches, and looked pale.

Of course, this would not necessarily be the case for everyone, since part of my problem is that I'm allergic to soy, peanuts and other member of the legume family, which is a staple in vegetarian diets.

But I've also read reports on yeast infections that show a link between vegetarianism and increased susceptibility to fungus. That is, unless you're doing it right and keeping your protein level at the right level for your body's requirements, the yeast can grow from the imbalance and the oversupply of carbohydrates.

After trying many different types of diets, the one that works best for me is one that focuses on:

- poultry

- fish

- occasionally beef

- non-legume vegetables

- some nuts and seeds like sesame and flax

- olive oil

Without realizing it, I eventually became aware after doing lots of reading that this was also known as a "caveman diet" or "Paleolithic diet" because of what archaeological research shows our original ancestors ate: seafood, game and vegetation (see the Resources chapter for reference and more details). It makes rational sense to me: this is what they ate because that's what there was to eat! Humans didn't start cultivating grains and livestock's milk on a regular basis until about 10,000 years ago. That sounds like a long time until you realize that humans have been around for at least 4 million years (and that numbers seems to keep getting longer with each new discovery and better methods of carbon dating).

So, our bodies, the ones we are using right now, evolved during at least 99% of our DNA's history of exposure to the food that was most readily available. Maybe there were some groups of people who only had exposure to vegetation for long periods of time and they created the gene that some people have now who don't tolerate meat well, same with some groups who had plentiful game but were not near coasts with seafood and maybe their descendants are the ones allergic to fish.

Impossible to say for sure, but a couple of things seem obvious: no people had heavy exposure to carbohydrates. Even fruits were sparse, seasonal and not in the well-cultivated, custom made, sugared up varieties we see in supermarkets today. They were small, hard, and fibrous—almost more like vegetables. When sugar was introduced to Europe around the 1500s from the newly discovered West Indies, the few wealthy people who could afford it, like Queen Elizabeth I, lost their teeth to it as it was such a foreign substance to our bodies. (A similarly harmful substance discovered in that same period was tobacco: we didn't evolve inhaling burning leaves either).

If we had evolved in the landscape of Willy Wonka's chocolate factory, where the streams are flowing melted chocolate and lollipops grow on bushes, then I'm sure that's what our bodies, ie, the DNA of any gene pool that made it this far through evolution, would thrive on. But we didn't.

I think that's why, with overwhelming frequency and consistency, the recommended diet for healing almost *any* kind of ailment is fresh, organic fish, meat, vegetables, seeds and their oils, and lots of water. No sugar and grains: maybe some gluten-free ones like buckwheat (which is actually a seed, not a grain) and brown rice (also not technically a grain). There is nothing mysterious about this diet: it's just not the one we have become accustomed to, especially during the last fifty years. The only slight matters in dispute seem to be what percentage each should carry in a specific diet for a specific purpose, or the merit of one particular food versus other, but the overall message was unmistakable to me at the time I discovered the diet that would cure my skin.

Another type of diet similar to the "caveman diet" is the anti-inflammation diet and its variants, like Dr Perricone's. They have become popular in the last couple of years as a treatment for the effects of aging on the skin and arthritis. It also focuses on organic poultry, fish, oils and vegetables, but gets more specific on the types by emphasizing the recent finding on the anti-inflammatory effects of the omega-3 component found in salmon and flaxseed. The only significant difference between these types of diet and the type I went on to inhibit candida is fruit.

And to go in an even more popular direction, the recent success of other low carb diets like The South Beach Diet, created by a doctor, used by millions and no significantly dangerous side effects found, gives further credence to the idea that millions of years of evolution have set up us perfectly to be able to facilitate health with some kind of combination of lean protein and produce. Even Oprah's diet guidelines on her website advise an emphasis on lean protein and green vegetables for two weeks, with *no* grains and only two servings of fruit per day.

For those of us who may have excess yeast, we just have to take it that one extra step that is so hard to stumble up on by accident: abstaining from fruits, starches and other sugars for awhile to compensate for the years of letting them build up.

6

The Diet and Recovery: Stages and Timing

There are six stages to the diet—each is one week long:

1. Week 1: Preparation

2. Week 2: Starting the Diet

3. Week 3: Continue the Diet; Round One of Natural Anti-Fungals

4. Week 4: Continue the Diet; Round Two of Natural Anti-Fungals

5. Week 5: Continue the Diet; Round Three of Natural Anti-Fungals

6. Week 6: Evaluate, Ease off the Diet and Curb any Inflammation

A note about the timing: these are guidelines only, based on what worked for *me*. It's not a science (yet), and I'm not a nutritionist. For your personal case, you may need more or less time at each stage, and you should check with your doctor—though be prepared to meet with skepticism about the entire anti-fungal approach to curing eczema. What you might want your doctor's blessing on, though, is a confirmation that there's nothing in this plan that will *harm* you. As long as he agrees on that, then hopefully you can carry on and see if there's something in it that will help you.

7

Week 1: Preparing for the Diet

There are three goals for the week before the diet to help clear out and prepare your system, so the actual diet won't be such an abrupt change for your system. It's already under enough stress: the idea is to gently ease into it. The first two are fairly standard—I'm sure you've seen them in other health programs and especially in detoxification plans:

- drink a full 10 to 12 glasses of purified water per day: aim for one per hour

- gradually cut down on caffeine until you're at one cup per day

- don't eat any food or drink for which you've ever seen an advertisement

The last one requires some explanation. "Don't eat or drink anything that appears in advertisements" is something I heard someone in the food industry say once casually, but it actually has a deep meaning when you think of advertising's impact on our grocery shopping habits.

Anything for sale is theoretically being sold at a profit, and then to buy commercial advertising on top of that is obviously very expensive. So, to make that profit, the item must then be sold at very high prices, which the market might not support, or use very cheap ingredients and manufacturing processes, like adding preservatives and sugars.

The one exception may be bottled water. But even that could be produced much more inexpensively and just as well at home with a basic water filtration system in a water jug in the refrigerator or on the kitchen sink tap.

I used to think oatmeal was another exception. But then I noticed that all the ads I saw on TV and even in print for never for the pure, plain kind: they were for the flavored ones with all that extra sugar added.

Then there are ads for orange juice, flavored yogurt, and soy products. Aren't these good for you? No, no and no. Not if you are trying to heal your skin. If you have no significant health problems, they may be just fine. But they tend to be loaded with sugar and fermentation or mold by-products. The ideal plan is for you to clear them out of your system for the duration of this diet then gradually be able to return to them by trying them one by one. By then, if you're like me, much of your taste for them will have diminished and some will actually taste foul to you. For example, I used to love croissants: I never saw a baked good I didn't like. But I've been on the maintenance stage of this diet for so long now, that when I saw a plate full of croissants at the office the other day, they truly looked like plastic to me: and that's what I know they'd taste like compared to what I now consider to be "real" food I had already had for breakfast.

On this diet, even though there are the occasional exceptions, I use this advertisement guideline to help make the choices easier. It also helped me become more aware of what I'm eating and where it came from. A similar guideline that many nutritionists use is "shop around the perimeter of the grocery store," meaning against the walls where the coolers are. (Not the beer though!) This means that the focus should be on fresh produce, fish, and poultry—but the problem is that there's a lot of other goodies intermingled now in those same areas in most groceries, so the increasing awareness I bring to the non-advertising principle helps me sort through them.

8

Week 2 to 5: The Diet

There are six stages and weeks to this diet and this is the second to fifth ones, so four weeks in all, as summarized below. It's short and simple—not easy, but simple.

Week 2: Start the Diet

The main goal of this week is to continue drinking lots of water, cut out caffeine (if you were really hooked on it like I was, try tapering off by just drinking green jasmine tea for the first couple of days), smoking, alcohol, and any other obvious toxins (decrease any medications if your doctor will allow it temporarily), eat only certain foods as listed below, organic if possible, and avoid certain foods.

After the first few days, you may experience, which I did, a temporary worsening of symptoms that may last for about a week. As the yeasts start to die, they release toxins that affect you. You may feel like you have the flu, you may experience cravings for carbs (which is probably the yeast talking, to try to get you to feed them so they can stay around in your system). The best thing to do is drink plenty of water, do deep breathing, take at least one half-hour walk per day, do some light stretching and yoga, and persist with the diet.

Week 3: Continue the Diet; Round One of Natural Anti-Fungals

The exact same diet: just add Pau D'Arco tea (can usually be found in any health food store, some drug stores, or online), three cups a day.

The idea is to introduce and rotate three different anti-fungals into your diet during the three main weeks of the diet, to weaken the yeast further, then kill it off, after the initial diet preparation period has weakened it. Yeast is very adaptable, however, and can take many different forms, so that is why you have to attack it with a new substance after a few days before it has much of a chance to mutate.

It's made from the bark of a South American tree and has a mild anti-fungal effect. This will ease you into the week where a significant amount of yeast should be weakening and leaving your system. Keep drinking lots of water and vegetables to flush them out of you.

The other reason I chose this for the beginning of the diet is to help give you something to replace any tea or coffee fix you may be missing. Not that this herb tea tastes like regular tea, but at least it's something, and I keep hearing that you can never actually get rid of or quit a bad habit: you can only replace it with something else.

That said, dandelion root tea does taste quite a bit like coffee in my opinion. Of any of the coffee substitutes out there, this seems closest, especially the roasted root type. It tastes like strong, bitter coffee with a black pepper edge. You can add stevia to sweeten it. Dandelion is a natural diuretic and good for the liver and kidneys, so is an excellent beverage to drink for the duration of the diet.

Week 4: Continue the Diet; Round Two of Natural Anti-Fungals

The exact same diet as the previous week: but stop the Pau D'Arco tea and eat a clove of fresh garlic twice a day with a bit of olive oil and parsley to control any odor. I wouldn't worry too much about it—parsley and oil are the main ingredients in many of the most effective bad breath capsules. And I think it was Dr Andrew Weil, the alternative medicine authority, who said something to the effect of, "if you think you smell, you will; if you don't, you won't," which is strangely true.

The point is that garlic is any extremely strong anti-fungal, has no known side effects, has many other natural health benefits as well, and is cheap and plentiful. That's why I chose it for my regime, and it worked.

The other point is that yes, it does have to be raw. And recently raw too: don't buy those pre-minced jars of garlic. Buy it fresh, slice it up, then eat it off a spoon with the oil and parsley, or mix it with a bit of salad. The active substance that kills the fungus is only released when the clove is crushed and the biochemicals mix, so it should be chewed first, then swallowed.

It makes sense when you think of how garlic, and so many other vegetables which is probably why most have some kind of anti-fungal properties in the raw, protect themselves from insects while growing. Bugs can probably only get so far before being turned off.

That said, a similar warning for humans: raw garlic may sting your mouth at first. It did mine, because I had oral thrush—but in a way it was good because it made me realize how badly I needed it, that it was working, and it was just a temporary stinging. Now I can eat it and it doesn't bother me at all: that also shows me how far I've come in the healing process. But just try a little bit a first, then gradually build up if it bothers you.

Week 5: Continue the Diet; Round Three of Natural Anti-Fungals

The exact same diet as the previous weeks: but replace garlic with grapefruit seed extract.

Not to be confused with grape seed extract, the one you want is derived from the core of the seed of the citrus fruit. It has a very bitter taste (you've probably noticed by now the paradoxical trend of bitter foods being good for us, sweet being usually bad), but you only need a few drops diluted into one glass of water three times a day to be effective.

Like garlic, grapefruit seed extract is strong, cheap, no known side effects and can be found in many health food stores or online. One bottle will last you a long time since you only need a few drops per day.

9

The Diet: Foods to Eat and Avoid

Foods to Eat:

- fish, especially coldwater oily fish like salmon, tuna, halibut, cod, sole, herring, trout and other whitefish

- chicken, turkey, duck, quail, lamb

- extra virgin cold-pressed olive oil, flaxseed oil and sesame oil

- coconut: oil, cream, milk and fresh meat

- raw almonds and almond butter

- flaxseed meal

- sesame seeds and butter (tahini); pumpkin seeds and butter

- fresh or frozen vegetables such as kale, spinach, cooked onion and garlic (will move on to raw in the next week's diet), Brussels sprouts, cabbage, radish, broccoli, cauliflower, turnip, leek, mustard greens, celery, cucumber

- fresh herbs like parsley, cilantro, dill, oregano, mint, rosemary, thyme, sage, basil, ginger

- sea salt with a light hand

- fruit: avocado, lemon and lime

- beverages: water, dandelion root tea, lemon and lime juice, fresh ginger tea

- sweetener: stevia

Foods to Avoid:

- no sugar or anything sweet in any form except for stevia: no dextrose, lactose, maple syrup, saccharine, aspartame, maltose, manitol, sorbitol, sucralose, brown sugar, molasses, raw sugar, honey

- no table salt, because believe it or not, most brands contain sugar (check the label)—I told this to a doctor once who had just appeared as a guest on a health show on TV: he didn't realize this fact and was floored; you can use a bit of sea salt instead

- no dairy: this includes all cheese, milk, yogurt, cream and whey

- no mushrooms, carrots, peas, other sweet or starchy vegetables like peppers, tomatoes, squash, corn, parsnip and potatoes

- no nuts except almonds; this includes peanuts, soy, and other legumes like beans or lentils (many nuts contain mold which feeds the yeast and burdens your system, especially peanuts, pistachios, and Brazil nuts)

- no grains and starches: no wheat, oats, rye, barley, rice, or corn (some gluten-free grains like rice, millet, amaranth and quinoa can eventually be added back as symptoms improve—corn is gluten-free but hard to digest, often moldy, and a common allergen, so it is best to avoid as long as possible)

- no fermented products like vinegar, condiments like relish, tofu, or yeast ingredients (including vitamins with yeast); no smoked or preserved meat or fish

- no dried fruit, meat or herbs initially

- no coffee, tea, chocolate, pure cocoa or soda, even if decaffeinated

Controversial Foods That I Tried, Then Avoided:

These are allowed in some anti-fungal diets I've seen, but not in others. I going on the premise that a skin infection of yeast may be tougher to get rid of than an infection in other common areas, like the stomach, based on what a doctor told me once about a bacterial staphylococcus infection on the skin requiring stronger antibiotics for a longer duration, and based on my own experience with curing it once, then having a relapse that was much harder to clean up.

So, I'm erring on the side of caution here by not including them in the "Foods to Eat" section, but these are probably among some of the first you can consider adding back into your diet after symptoms have cleared and stabilized for about a month:

- beef, veal, pork and shellfish: many diets cite the high acidity of beef as a reason to exclude it; I personally tolerate it well but don't eat it often—organic beef about once a week. Apparently pork and shellfish carry a lot of toxins

- eggs: I say leave them off to start and avoid them for at least three weeks, then try one to see if you're allergic to it

- yogurt: no—it's either got dairy, soy, or sugar in it, and you can get the good bacteria from taking an acidophilus supplement instead

- tomatoes: fresh should be ok to add back early, unless you find you're allergic to them, but avoid canned tomatoes in any form for as long as possible, as they're said to be made with a high percentage of tomatoes that have gone moldy

- cashew nuts: I personally love them, but are high in carbs compared to most nuts: save until the post-diet maintenance phase

- roasted nuts and seeds: add moderate amounts back in early, like roasted almonds, macadamias, sunflower, pecan and walnuts if you can tolerate them; raw is still best for most nuts, though I've read that some roasting can prevent mold, and I've recently started to be able to taste mold in raw sunflower seeds, so I'm hoping that more conclusive evidence will soon be available

- apples and cranberries: I know these are on many detox and anti-candida diets, but for me they were too sweet and I wouldn't feel well after eating them

- green tea: it contains caffeine, so it should be avoided for at least the duration of the diet

10

Recipes

I think it was Nigella Lawson, the British chef, who said of one of her preparations something like, "this is assembled, rather than cooked." The same could be said for most of my meal ideas, below. I'm no great cook, but found that these were my staples during the diet, most of which I just threw together by mixing whatever foods were allowed.

I list some websites, some of which have tons of recipes, at the end of the book—just with the caveat that many of the sites have varying strictness to the diet, ie, some allow cocoa, some dairy, etc, so please adjust their recipes accordingly if you have eczema, as from my own experience this condition calls for *the* strictest interpretation of the diet.

Almond Cereal

½ cup sliced almonds
2 tsp whole grain flax seeds soaked overnight, or unsoaked ground meal
3 tbsp coconut cream or milk, fresh or canned
Stevia powder to taste, for sweetness

Just mix together in a bowl. Another option, if you don't have or like coconut or want it hot, is to substitute warm water and let it soak for a minute. The only problem with that is that the beneficial oil in the flax is very heat-sensitive, so it's better to not overheat it. The whole flax seeds have a nuttier taste than the ground meal: they need to be pre-soaked but it's worth it.

Omega-3 Coleslaw

4 cups shredded green and/or purple cabbage
(or one package of prepared cabbage from the grocery: pick out the pieces of carrot)
½ cup chopped celery
¼ cup chopped cilantro
Juice of half a fresh lemon
2 tbsp olive oil
2 tsp flaxseed meal
Celery seed: a dash
Stevia: a few drops or one envelope powder
Sea salt: a dash

Just mix together in a big bowl. This tastes amazingly good—something about the whole is better than the sum of its parts. I got the idea after hearing from a friend who was in the Marines about how much sugar there is in coleslaw, which he found out after helping to make huge batches for the troops. I always thought it was just as healthy as eating plain vegetables. In this, we substitute stevia instead.

This can also be a good base for a salad for which you can throw in chopped chicken or tuna. Sometimes I substitute some coconut cream for the oil, to make it more like creamy coleslaw or tuna salad.

Leek Soup

1 large leek, well cleaned and chopped
2 sliced garlic cloves
Sea salt to taste
4 cups water

Bring water to a boil; add ingredients; simmer for thirty minutes. This is another dish that is deceptively simple and great-tasting—I never thought it would be very good, but now I'm hooked on it. It's also a natural diuretic and makes you feel much better when you have a cold.

Sesame Salmon Spinach Salad

1 can or 6 oz of baked salmon
2 cups chopped spinach
1 tbsp sesame oil
Toasted sesame seeds
Chopped green onions to taste

Just mix together in a big bowl!

Lemon Garlic Chicken

2 chicken breasts, or 4 thighs or drumsticks
½ a fresh lemon
4 garlic cloves
Fresh rosemary and/or thyme
Sea salt

Preheat the oven to 350 degrees F. Spread the chicken out in a roasting pan, squirt lemon juice on it, sprinkle with herbs and salt, throw garlic in the pan; cook for about one hour.

Sage Stuffing

1 large onion, chopped
1 pound ground turkey
¼ cup olive oil
1 cup celery, chopped
Sea salt to taste
2 tbsp minced sage
½ cup fresh parsley, chopped
1 tsp fennel seeds
2 cups almond meal

Preheat oven to 350 degrees F. Grease a small pan with olive oil. Sauté all the ingredients in a skillet on the stove until cooked. Transfer to the baking dish; bake 20 minutes, take out and mix, then another 20 minutes or until browned.

Beef and Broccoli

1 large onion, chopped
1 clove garlic, chopped
½ pound stewing beef or hamburger
1 crown of broccoli, chopped
Sea salt to taste

I find I don't miss soy sauce when I can brown some sautéed onions instead. Soy sauce is mostly salt anyway, plus some kind of caramel color and flavor that is similar to caramelized onions. Brown the onion, garlic, salt and beef together, then add the broccoli on top, cover and let simmer for about 10 minutes until broccoli is done.

Ginger Cabbage

1 large onion
About 1 inch of ginger root, minced
Half a head of cabbage

Sauté together until cabbage is tender. This is quite a different taste with cooked cabbage compared to the raw cabbage of the coleslaw recipe. The ginger gives it an Asian aroma, and is great for settling your stomach and improving digestion.

Almond Macaroons

½ cup raw almond butter
1 cup dried unsweetened coconut
Stevia: a few drops of liquid or 1 envelope powder
Vanilla: pure extract with no sugar or alcohol, or fresh vanilla bean

Mix together in a bowl, adding enough coconut so the butter stops sticking; roll into 1 inch balls. No baking required!

Coconut Ice Cream

1 can of coconut cream or milk
Stevia: a few drops or 1 envelope
Vanilla: pure extract with no sugar or alcohol, or fresh vanilla bean
Lemon zest (optional)

Open the can and pour or scoop the top half of the contents in one bowl; set aside the bottom half (save for milk for cereal or coleslaw). Mix the other ingredients into the bowl and refrigerate (not freeze) for a few hours until firm.

Snacks

- vegetables with tahini and garlic for a dip

- sliced avocado sprinkled with salt and green onions

- a handful of almonds

- lemon juice, stevia and fresh ginger slices, with hot or cold water; cold, it tastes like ginger ale; hot is great for congestion

11

Week 6: Evaluate, Ease Off the Diet, and Curb Inflammation

Your skin should be clear: if not, but you see improvement, don't worry. If you've had eczema for years and years like I did, one round of the diet may not be sufficient, but is the necessary beginning.

What I did at this point, during my fight against the relapse of my condition, where one round on the diet wasn't enough but I could see that it was working, was I went back on cortisone creams: it cleared it up immediately, and stayed that way, unlike the times I'd used cortisone before the diet.

That's what made me think the cortisone just can't work with you unless you create a good working environment for it first by clearing the yeast out of your system. Yeast is an *interferer*.

So try the cortisone, then another round of the diet if necessary. I've read that you need to be on the diet for at least half the time that you were ill, since symptoms started appearing. But it didn't take nearly that long for me, even with life-long, stubborn eczema, so I hope it won't for you as well. As of the time of the writing of this book, I'm about six months along to going a full year without fruit or grains, then I'll try them again.

Adding to Your Diet:

By now you will probably notice that most of your cravings for sweets and carbs are gone. I strongly believe that is the basis for the epidemic in overeating today: it's not willpower, it's the yeast!

Foods taste better now and you should be able to taste the molds in foods you used to eat all the time without realizing it.

Add back to your diet: dried herbs, especially turmeric and cinnamon, which is an anti-inflammatory and recommended as a natural aid to many health issues.

You can add those two to many of the recipes you were making during the diet and they will perk them up immensely.

Also add, every other day (leaving a day in between to evaluate), *small* portions in generally this order of organic:

- beef

- brown rice

- veal

- low-mold nuts like walnuts, pecans, hazelnuts

- grapefruit

- millet

- green beans

- tomatoes

- squash, parsnip, raw carrots

- cranberries

- amaranth

- eggs

- quinoa

- new potatoes

- apples

- soy beans

- green tea

- other items as you like

Make sure to watch your reactions closely: note any stomach upset and difference in bowel movements, as I found those usually preceded skin flare-ups by a day or two.

12

Maintenance, Supplements and Tips

1. Dry out your environment. I don't think that humidity necessarily causes eczema and candida growth, but it can exacerbate it. Try to have any mold or mildew in your home eliminated. Get a dehumidifier: I did and it makes a big difference—it's not as expensive as an air conditioner.

2. Note your food sensitivities as you sense them, then go to an allergist and have allergy skin tests done to see if you are allergic to foods you didn't know about. I was surprised to find out I was allergic to soy and wheat. Cutting those out allowed me to finally heal. The allergist also started me on shots for cat, dog, hay fever and dust mite allergies, and those seem to be helping: plus I know to avoid them in the meantime, and that has helped my skin too.

3. The daily supplements I used were: extra calcium and vitamin C, magnesium, a yeast-free multivitamin, acidophilus probiotics (the refrigerated kind) in all their recommended doses; plus the herbs that I was already fairly familiar with, like ginger root, dandelion root, milk thistle, turmeric—but there are many more listed in the websites below. I just didn't get around to trying them all, and my skin was in such bad shape that I didn't want to risk taking something that might be harmful to it, so in the book I've only mentioned what I've actually experienced.

4. Try a few different forms of stevia: the liquid is good for cooking or on a salad. You just need a few drops. But it has a bit of flavor that's hard to describe: kind of carroty. So I don't use it in beverages—I used the little stevia pills or envelopes of powder.

5. I threw out my "natural" toothpaste when I found it had sorbitol and sodium lauryl hydrate in it. Those are not good for this diet. I finally

found another one that uses stevia—but it also has honey in it! Did I miss something, or are we not supposed to use sugar on our teeth? So I started using a bit of diluted hydrogen peroxide and sometimes baking soda. Those work great. My teeth are bright white, and I recently went to the dentist who said everything looks perfect.

6. I also got a sodium lauryl hydrate-free shampoo at a health food store. I don't know for sure if it's bad for my skin, but with what you can find about it on the internet, it doesn't look good.

7. After bathing, which I still do twice a day and makes my skin feel better, I make sure to dry creases well, especially between my toes, and often use a hairdryer to make sure they're dry. Moist areas support fungus.

8. I also used a regular, over the counter, anti-fungal cream for athlete's foot on my feet, ankles, and other stubborn areas. You can tell how stubborn fungus is in your system just by reading the directions to the cream: use for four weeks! And that's for someone who doesn't have a serious systemic infection. A minimum of four weeks seems to be how long it takes for yeast to go through the stages of elimination, but six was necessary for me.

9. There's also a complicating factor called Leaky Gut Syndrome which often comes along with candida overgrowth: I am now starting to treat myself for that by continuing to stay on the diet, with a few additions like brown rice and beef, and will start taking L-Glutamine to help it heal. There is more information on this on many of the websites I've listed in the Resources section.

Appendix

Internet Resources

The Skin Cure Diet Website
www.skincurediet.com

This is my website with a summary of the book and links to other resources. I'll post updates, frequently-asked questions and answers, and news whenever they're available, so please check in often.

Karen Tripp: Candida Recovery
www.geocities.com/HotSprings/4966/index.html

Thanks out to Karen, whose site was one of the first, if not the first, I stumbled upon when realizing I had yeast and not just bad skin and allergies. She has her full story, her advice, and tons of recipes. Her recovery was very swift compared to most, so please recognize that she may already have been in very good health (ie, she's young and a dancer) before starting her regime. Also, she did not have any major skin problem; so, I would start strict at first, then move on to her recipes, etc, as your condition permits—same advice goes with the rest of these sites, below.

Shirley's Wellness Café
www.shirleys-wellness-cafe.com

Good sections on candida, eczema and a "healing crisis" and why we often get worse before we get better; the stages and how to tell the difference

The Wellness Guru
www.wellnessguru.com/wellness_candida-2.htm

Interesting take on the effect of the acidity of different foods and their effect on candida overgrowth. Also tables showing different foods to eat at five different stages of recovery.

Slow Oxidizer Eating Plan
www.drlwilson.com/Articles/slow%20diet.htm

This article fascinates me because it's a low carb diet but has nothing to do with candida, just a doctor-recommended all-purpose healing diet for optimal digestion. Note the emphasis on meat and vegetables.

Paleolithic Diet versus Vegetarianism: What Was Humanity's Original, Natural Diet?
www.beyondveg.com/nicholson-w/hb/hb-interview1a.shtml

Interesting, detailed interview with a researcher on this subject.

Paleofood
www.paleofood.com

Tons of recipes that focus on meat, fish and vegetables.

Nutritionhelp
www.nutritionhelp.com/candida.php

Good detail, explanation and FAQs on candida by a nutritionist. She goes into the fibromyalgia connection and die-off reactions.

Mold and Diet
www.naturalhealthweb.com/articles/b2.html

The effects of mold on diet and the many different symptoms that it can cause.

Candida FAQ 2.0
web.archive.org/web/20020802012431/www.infosky.net/~alexmi/candida.htm

Very detailed.

978-0-595-35883-0
0-595-35883-7

Printed in the United States
70682LV00004B/379